Date:_____

TIME	FOOD	
	TOTAL	

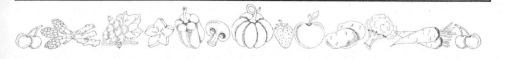

Notes

Date:_____   I Feel 😊 😣 😐

TIME	FOOD	CALORIES
	TOTAL	

Notes

Date:_____ I Feel 😊 😟 😐

TIME	FOOD	CALORIES
	TOTAL	

Notes

Date:_____   I Feel 😊 😧 😐

TIME	FOOD	CALORIES
	TOTAL	

Notes

Date:_____   I Feel 😊 😦 😐

TIME	FOOD	CALORIES
	TOTAL	

Notes

Date:_____ I Feel 😊 😟 😊

TIME	FOOD	CALORIES
	TOTAL	

Notes

Date:_____   I Feel 😊 😣 😐

TIME	FOOD	CALORIES
	TOTAL	

Notes

Date:_____   I Feel 😊 😟 😐

TIME	FOOD	CALORIES
	TOTAL	

Notes

Date:_____   I Feel 😊 🙁 😐

TIME	FOOD	CALORIES
	TOTAL	

Notes

Date:_____   I Feel 😊 😣 😐

TIME	FOOD	CALORIES
	TOTAL	

Notes

Date:_____ I Feel 😊 🙁 😐

TIME	FOOD	CALORIES
	TOTAL	

Notes

Date:_____ I Feel 🙂 🙁 🙂

TIME	FOOD	CALORIES
	TOTAL	

Notes

Date:_____   I Feel 😊 😞 😐

TIME	FOOD	CALORIES
	TOTAL	

Notes

Date:_____   I Feel 😊 🙁 😐

TIME	FOOD	CALORIES
	TOTAL	

Notes

Date:_____   I Feel 😊 🙁 😐

TIME	FOOD	CALORIES
	TOTAL	

Notes

Date:_____   I Feel 😊 😖 😐

TIME	FOOD	CALORIES
	TOTAL	

Notes

Date:_____   I Feel 😊 😟 😐

TIME	FOOD	CALORIES
	TOTAL	

Notes

Date:_____   I Feel 😊 😞 😐

TIME	FOOD	CALORIES
	TOTAL	

Notes

Date:_____ I Feel 😊 😞 😐

TIME	FOOD	CALORIES
	TOTAL	

Notes

Date:_____   I Feel 😊 😞 😐

TIME	FOOD	CALORIES
	TOTAL	

Notes

Date:_____   I Feel 😊 🙁 😐

TIME	FOOD	CALORIES
	TOTAL	

Notes

Date:_____   I Feel 😊 😟 😐

TIME	FOOD	CALORIES
	TOTAL	

Notes

Date:_____ I Feel 😊 😩 😐

TIME	FOOD	CALORIES
	TOTAL	

Notes

Date:_____   I Feel 😊 🙁 😐

TIME	FOOD	CALORIES
	TOTAL	

Notes

Date:_____   I Feel 😊 😟 😐

TIME	FOOD	CALORIES
	TOTAL	

Notes

Date:_____   I Feel 😊 😣 😐

TIME	FOOD	CALORIES
	TOTAL	

Notes

Date:_____   I Feel 😊 🙁 😐

TIME	FOOD	CALORIES
	TOTAL	

Notes

Date:_____   I Feel 😊 😖 😐

TIME	FOOD	CALORIES
	TOTAL	

Notes

Date:_____   I Feel 😊 😖 😐

TIME	FOOD	CALORIES
	TOTAL	

Notes

Date:_____   I Feel 😊 😞 😐

TIME	FOOD	CALORIES
	TOTAL	

Notes

Date:_____   I Feel 😊 😟 😐

TIME	FOOD	CALORIES
	TOTAL	

Notes

Date:_____   I Feel 😊 😞 😐

TIME	FOOD	CALORIES
	TOTAL	

Notes

Date:_____ I Feel 😊 🙁 😐

TIME	FOOD	CALORIES
	TOTAL	

Notes

Date:_____ I Feel 🙂 🙁 😐

TIME	FOOD	CALORIES
	TOTAL	

Notes

Date:_____ I Feel 😊 😟 😐

TIME	FOOD	CALORIES
	TOTAL	

Notes

Date:_____   I Feel 😊 😟 😐

TIME	FOOD	CALORIES
	TOTAL	

Notes

Date:_____   I Feel 😊 😟 😐

TIME	FOOD	CALORIES
	TOTAL	

Notes

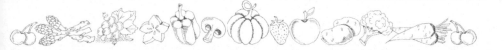

Date:_____   I Feel 😊 😣 😐

TIME	FOOD	CALORIES
	TOTAL	

Notes

Date:_____ I Feel 🙂 🙁 😐

TIME	FOOD	CALORIES
	TOTAL	

Notes

Date:_____   I Feel 😊 😟 😐

TIME	FOOD	CALORIES
	TOTAL	

Notes

Date:_____   I Feel 😊 🙁 😐

TIME	FOOD	CALORIES
	TOTAL	

Notes

Date:_____   I Feel 😊 😞 😐

TIME	FOOD	CALORIES
	TOTAL	

Notes

Date:_____ I Feel 😊 😞 😐

TIME	FOOD	CALORIES
	TOTAL	

Notes

Date:_____ I Feel 😊 😟 😐

TIME	FOOD	CALORIES
	TOTAL	

Notes

Date:_____ I Feel 😊 😔 😐

TIME	FOOD	CALORIES
	TOTAL	

Notes

Date:_____   I Feel 😊 😟 😐

TIME	FOOD	CALORIES
	TOTAL	

Notes

Date:_____ I Feel 😊 😟 😐

TIME	FOOD	CALORIES
	TOTAL	

Notes

Date:_____   I Feel 😊 ☹ 😐

TIME	FOOD	CALORIES
	TOTAL	

Notes

Date:_____ I Feel 😊 😟 😐

TIME	FOOD	CALORIES
	TOTAL	

Notes

Date:_____   I Feel 😊 😞 😐

TIME	FOOD	CALORIES
	TOTAL	

Notes

Date:_____ I Feel 😊 😣 😐

TIME	FOOD	CALORIES
	TOTAL	

Notes

Date:_____   I Feel 😊 😟 😐

TIME	FOOD	CALORIES
	TOTAL	

Notes

Date:_____   I Feel 😊 😞 😐

TIME	FOOD	CALORIES
	TOTAL	

Notes

Date:_____ I Feel 😊 😖 😐

TIME	FOOD	CALORIES
	TOTAL	

Notes

Date:_____ I Feel 😊 😞 😐

TIME	FOOD	CALORIES
	TOTAL	

Notes

Date:_____ I Feel 😊 😞 😐

TIME	FOOD	CALORIES
	TOTAL	

Notes

Date:_____ I Feel 😊 😞 😐

TIME	FOOD	CALORIES
	TOTAL	

Notes

Date:_____   I Feel 😊 😖 😐

TIME	FOOD	CALORIES
	TOTAL	

Notes

Date:_____ I Feel 😊 😟 😐

TIME	FOOD	CALORIES
	TOTAL	

Notes

Date:_____   I Feel 😊 🙁 😐

TIME	FOOD	CALORIES
	TOTAL	

Notes

Date:_____ I Feel 🙂 🙁 😐

TIME	FOOD	CALORIES
	TOTAL	

Notes

Date:_____ I Feel 😊 😟 😐

TIME	FOOD	CALORIES
	TOTAL	

Notes

Date:_____   I Feel 😊 😣 😐

TIME	FOOD	CALORIES
	TOTAL	

Notes

Date:_____   I Feel 😊 😞 😐

TIME	FOOD	CALORIES
	TOTAL	

Notes

Date:_____   I Feel 😊 😠 😐

TIME	FOOD	CALORIES
	TOTAL	

Notes

Date:_____ I Feel 😊 😞 😐

TIME	FOOD	CALORIES
	TOTAL	

Notes

Date:_____   I Feel 🙂 🙁 😐

TIME	FOOD	CALORIES
	TOTAL	

Notes

Date:_____ I Feel 😊 🙁 😐

TIME	FOOD	CALORIES
	TOTAL	

Notes

Date:_____ I Feel 🙂 🙁 😐

TIME	FOOD	CALORIES
	TOTAL	

Notes

Date:_____   I Feel 😊 😣 😐

TIME	FOOD	CALORIES
	TOTAL	

Notes

Date:_____   I Feel 😊 🙁 😐

TIME	FOOD	CALORIES
	TOTAL	

Notes

Date:_____ I Feel 😊 😞 😐

TIME	FOOD	CALORIES
	TOTAL	

Notes

Date:_____   I Feel 😊 😠 😐

TIME	FOOD	CALORIES
	TOTAL	

Notes

Date:_____   I Feel :) :(:|

TIME	FOOD	CALORIES
	TOTAL	

Notes

Date:_____   I Feel 😊 😟 😐

TIME	FOOD	CALORIES
	TOTAL	

Notes

Date:_____   I Feel 😊 😣 😐

TIME	FOOD	CALORIES
	TOTAL	

Notes

Date:_____   I Feel 😊 🙁 😐

TIME	FOOD	CALORIES
	TOTAL	

Notes

Date:_____   I Feel 😊 🙁 😐

TIME	FOOD	CALORIES
	TOTAL	

Notes

Date:_____ I Feel 😊 😞 😐

TIME	FOOD	CALORIES
	TOTAL	

Notes

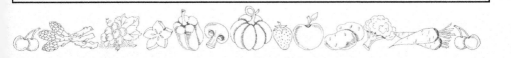

Date:_____   I Feel 😊 😞 😐

TIME	FOOD	CALORIES
	TOTAL	

Notes

Date:_____ I Feel 😊 😣 😐

TIME	FOOD	CALORIES
	TOTAL	

Notes

Date:_____

I Feel 😊 😦 😐

TIME	FOOD	CALORIES
	TOTAL	

Notes

Date:_____ I Feel 🙂 🙁 😐

TIME	FOOD	CALORIES
	TOTAL	

Notes

Date:_____ I Feel 😊 😞 😐

TIME	FOOD	CALORIES
	TOTAL	

Notes

Date:_____   I Feel 😊 😞 😐

TIME	FOOD	CALORIES
	TOTAL	

Notes

Date:_____   I Feel 😊 😞 😐

TIME	FOOD	CALORIES
	TOTAL	

Notes

Date:_____   I Feel 😊 😟 😐

TIME	FOOD	CALORIES
	TOTAL	

Notes

Date:_____   I Feel :) :(:|

TIME	FOOD	CALORIES
	TOTAL	

Notes

Date:_____   I Feel 😊 😞 😐

TIME	FOOD	CALORIES
	TOTAL	

Notes

Date:_____ I Feel 🙂 🙁 😐

TIME	FOOD	CALORIES
	TOTAL	

Notes

Date:_____   I Feel 😊 😞 😐

TIME	FOOD	CALORIES
	TOTAL	

Notes

*Date:*_____   *I Feel* 😊 😣 😐

TIME	FOOD	CALORIES
	TOTAL	

Notes

Date:_____   I Feel 😊 ☹️ 😐

TIME	FOOD	CALORIES
	TOTAL	

Notes

Date:_____   I Feel :) :(:|

TIME	FOOD	CALORIES
	TOTAL	

Notes

Date:_____   I Feel 😊 😖 😐

TIME	FOOD	CALORIES
	TOTAL	

Notes

Date:_____   I Feel 😊 😟 😐

TIME	FOOD	CALORIES
	TOTAL	

Notes

Date:_____   I Feel 😊 🙁 😐

TIME	FOOD	CALORIES
	TOTAL	

Notes

Date:_____ I Feel 😊 🙁 😐

TIME	FOOD	CALORIES
	TOTAL	

Notes

Date:_____   I Feel 😊 😞 😐

TIME	FOOD	CALORIES
	TOTAL	

Notes

Date:_____   I Feel 😊 😞 😐

TIME	FOOD	CALORIES
	TOTAL	

Notes

Date:_____   I Feel 😊 😟 😐

TIME	FOOD	CALORIES
	TOTAL	

Notes

Date:_____ I Feel 😊 😞 😐

TIME	FOOD	CALORIES
	TOTAL	

Notes

Date:_____ I Feel 😊 😟 😐

TIME	FOOD	CALORIES
	TOTAL	

Notes

Date:_____ I Feel 🙂 🙁 😐

TIME	FOOD	CALORIES
	TOTAL	

Notes

Date:_____   I Feel 😊 😟 😐

TIME	FOOD	CALORIES
	TOTAL	

Notes

Date:_____   *I Feel* 😊 😞 😐

TIME	FOOD	CALORIES
	TOTAL	

Notes

Date:_____   I Feel 😊 😖 😐

TIME	FOOD	CALORIES
	TOTAL	

Notes

Date:_____   I Feel 😊 😟 😐

TIME	FOOD	CALORIES
	TOTAL	

Notes

Date:_____ I Feel 🙂 🙁 😐

TIME	FOOD	CALORIES
	TOTAL	

Notes

Date:_____   I Feel 😊 😞 😐

TIME	FOOD	CALORIES
	TOTAL	

Notes

Date:_____   I Feel 😊 😟 😐

TIME	FOOD	CALORIES
	TOTAL	

Notes

Printed in Great Britain
by Amazon

76231526R00068